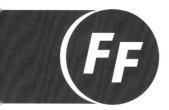

FAST FACTS

FF

Indispensable
Guides to
Clinical
Practice

Benign G̲ ̲ ̲ ̲ ̲ ̲ ̲ ̲
Disease

Second edition

John A Rock
James Robert McCord Professor
of Gynecology and Obstetrics,
Emory University School of Medicine,
Atlanta, Georgia, USA

R William Stones
Senior Lecturer, Obstetrics and Gynaecology,
University of Southampton,
Princess Anne Hospital, Southampton, UK

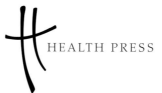

HEALTH PRESS

Oxford

Fast Facts – Benign Gynecological Disease
First published 1997
Reprinted 1998
Second edition November 2002

Text © 2002 John A Rock, R William Stones
© 2002 in this edition Health Press Limited
Health Press Limited, Elizabeth House, Queen Street, Abingdon,
Oxford OX14 3JR, UK
Tel: +44 (0)1235 523233
Fax: +44 (0)1235 523238

Fast Facts is a trade mark of Health Press Limited.

The publisher and the authors have made every effort to ensure the
accuracy of this book, but cannot accept responsibility for any errors
or omissions.

Registered names, trademarks, etc. used in this book, even when not
marked as such, are not to be considered unprotected by law.

A CIP catalogue record for this title is available from the British Library.

ISBN 1-903734-10-X

Rock, J (John) A
Fast Facts – Benign Gynecological Disease/
John A Rock, R William Stones

Illustrated by Dee McLean and Jane Fallows, London, UK.

Typeset by Zed, Oxford, UK.

Printed by Fine Print (Services) Ltd, Oxford, UK.

Glossary

Amenorrhea: abnormal cessation of menstruation

BV: bacterial vaginosis

Cervical ectropion: change in content of the vaginal cervix from squamous to columnar epithelium

Clue cells: vaginal epithelial cells coated with the pathogens responsible for bacterial vaginosis

CT: computerized tomography

D & C: dilatation (of the cervix) and curettage (of the endometrium)

DUB: dysfunctional uterine bleeding

Dysmenorrhea: pain associated with menstruation

Dyspareunia: difficult or painful coitus

Endometrial ablation: surgical removal of the endometrium

Endometriosis: presence of tissue histologically similar to endometrium outside the uterine cavity and the myometrium

Follicular phase: phase of the menstrual cycle during which the follicle is formed and the endometrium starts to proliferate

FSH: follicle-stimulating hormone, secreted by the pituitary gland

GnRH: gonadotropin-releasing hormone, produced by the hypothalamus

hCG: human chorionic gonadotropin, produced by the placenta during pregnancy

Hysteroscopy: direct visualization of the cervical canal and the uterine cavity

IUD: intrauterine device

Laparoscopy: endoscopic examination of the peritoneal cavity

Luteal phase: later stage of the menstrual cycle when the endometrium has fully developed

LH: luteinizing hormone, secreted by the pituitary gland

LH surge: sudden and large increase in the secretion of LH and FSH that occurs in the middle of the menstrual cycle

MRI: magnetic resonance imaging

Myomectomy: surgical removal of a fibroid

NSAIDs: non-steroidal anti-inflammatory drugs, used for pain relief

OC: oral contraceptive

Oligomenorrhea: infrequent menstruation

PCOS: polycystic ovary syndrome

PID: pelvic inflammatory disease, a condition in which the uterus, Fallopian tubes and ovaries are infected

PMS: premenstrual syndrome

S-CJ: the squamo-columnar junction between two epithelia

VVC: vulvovaginal candidiasis

Whiff test: smelling for the presence of anaerobic bacteria (associated with bacterial vaginosis) in the vaginal discharge. The 'whiff' is due to the release of amines on addition of potassium hydroxide (KOH)

Introduction

Benign gynecological disease and, in particular, menstrual disorders represent the main reason for patient referral to a gynecologist, reflecting a substantial workload for family physicians. Management of such conditions produces many challenges, and some of our patients are not best served either by their attending family physician or their gynecologist. The reasons for this are complex and reflect the large number of consultations, the complicated physiology of the reproductive cycle, the apparently poor efficacy of some medical treatments and the fact that the diseases are not seen as serious or life threatening. These diseases do, however, have significant impact on the lives of many women and can cause major problems at work and at home, especially in relationships with partners. The management of these disorders is usually simple, and it is the aim of this book to produce a clear blueprint for the family physician and non-specialized junior hospital doctor which they may use when dealing with benign gynecological disorders.

A brief review of the fundamental principles of reproductive physiology is included, as this is vital to the understanding of the pathogenesis of these disorders and the mechanisms through which a number of medical treatments work. Disorders of the menstrual cycle and their treatment are discussed in detail, as well as pelvic pain, which is regularly associated with menstruation and menstrual disorders. Pelvic pain is also one of the most common reasons for a patient to be referred to a gynecologist, and its management could be improved if certain basic principles were followed. Other topics associated with menstrual disorders are covered, including endometriosis and fibroids. The penultimate chapter deals with vaginitis, one of the most common gynecological conditions encountered by primary care practitioners.

Fast Facts – Benign Gynecological Disease provides up-to-date guidelines on the management of these disorders, together with a concise overview of physiology and diagnosis.

Reproductive physiology

Historic and social perspectives

The human female reproductive cycle is one of the most elegant examples of endocrinology in the animal kingdom. *Homo sapiens* is unusual in not having a breeding season and, together with some higher order primates, we are the only animals that menstruate.

Currently, a woman undergoes the earliest menarche and the latest menopause that the species has ever experienced; the average woman will experience 450 menstruations. The introduction of contraception has allowed fertility to be controlled, resulting in average family sizes of slightly less than two; women also tend to lactate for shorter periods. Historically this was not the case. When the species existed as hunter–gatherers, as exemplified today by the Kung tribe of South Africa, menarche occurred later and menopause earlier. It was common practice to lactate for 3 to 4 years, so allowing offspring to be spaced. As a result, a woman would have five or six children and, because of the amenorrhea of lactation, would only experience approximately 30 menstruations in her life.

In evolutionary terms, therefore, repeated exposure to menstruation is very recent and not the state in which biologically we should exist. This is important in our understanding of what constitutes a menstrual disorder. Demonstrable pathology may not be the cause of the problem but may reflect the degree of exposure to the phenomenon. However, this does not minimize the importance of the problem or diminish the need for successful treatment.

Endocrinology of the menstrual cycle

The interaction of the main hormones involved in the control of the menstrual cycle and the blood concentrations of those hormones during a typical 28-day cycle are shown in Figures 1.1 and 1.2.

Gonadotropin-releasing hormone (GnRH) is a small polypeptide produced by the hypothalamus. It flows through the pituitary portal

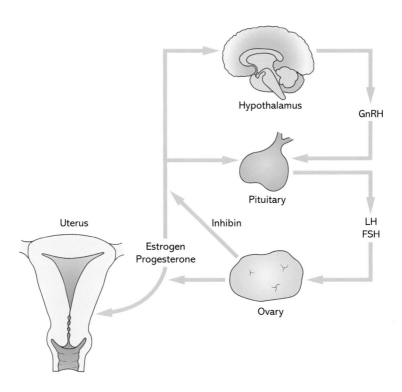

Figure 1.1 GnRH stimulates the release of LH and FSH which, in turn, stimulate estrogen and progesterone secretion, and follicular development. Estrogen initially has an inhibitory effect on gonadotropin secretion (negative feedback) but, later, high levels trigger the release of high levels of LH (positive feedback) which induce ovulation. Estrogen and progesterone stimulate endometrial proliferation in preparation for implantation.

system to stimulate the secretion of luteinizing hormone (LH) and follicle-stimulating hormone (FSH) from the pituitary gland. GnRH is released in pulses every 90 minutes and this pulsatile secretion is vital for continued reproductive cyclicity. Paradoxically, continuous secretion of the hormone leads to decreased stimulation of the pituitary. Manipulation of this mechanism has led to the development of GnRH agonists, important drugs in the treatment of benign gynecological disease. The secretion of GnRH is controlled by neurotransmitters from

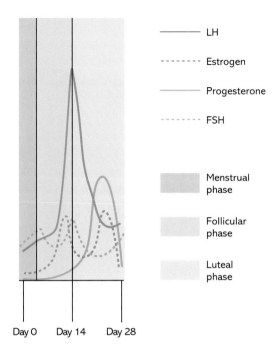

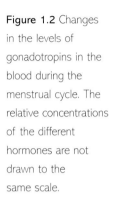

Figure 1.2 Changes in the levels of gonadotropins in the blood during the menstrual cycle. The relative concentrations of the different hormones are not drawn to the same scale.

the higher cerebral centers and by feedback of estrogen, progesterone and inhibin from the ovary.

LH and FSH are two glycoproteins secreted by the pituitary in response to a GnRH pulse and thus have a pulsatile pattern of secretion themselves. However, this pulsatile pattern is not essential for them to stimulate the ovary. During the follicular phase, LH and FSH stimulate the formation of the follicle, which is a cystic structure 2 cm in diameter found in the ovary and containing the oocyte. Under the influence of these hormones, the follicle secretes increasing amounts of estrogen.

At the middle of the cycle there is a sudden and large increase in the secretion of LH and FSH – the LH surge – which lasts 3 days. This massive endocrine signal changes the function of the oocyte which restarts meiotic division, and causes the follicle to rupture. This process is called ovulation and results in the extrusion of the oocyte into the fallopian tube. The ruptured follicle now changes into a structure called the corpus luteum, which secretes progesterone under the stimulation of LH. If no pregnancy results, the corpus luteum will start to degenerate.

LH and FSH are primarily controlled by the pulsatile secretion of GnRH; however, both estrogen and progesterone also exert control via the pituitary.

Estradiol is the main steroid hormone secreted by the developing follicle. It controls the growth of the endometrium in the follicular phase of the cycle, mainly by increasing the number of cells. Its secretion is controlled by LH and FSH.

Progesterone is the main steroid hormone produced by the corpus luteum. It changes the function of the glands in the endometrium, which have already been prepared by estrogen, so that the tissue is suitable for the implantation of the developing embryo which occurs 7 days after the LH surge. If the pregnancy does not implant and thus there is no secretion of human chorionic gonadotropin (hCG) from the trophoblast, the corpus luteum will start to decrease secretion of progesterone after the 7 days and menstruation will occur. It is the detection of hCG in the blood or urine which forms the basis of modern pregnancy tests.

Timing of the menstrual cycle

The current average ages of menarche and menopause are 13 and 51 years, respectively. Women are usually consistent with the length of their menstrual cycle over time, but considerable variability exists between individuals. The normal length of the follicular phase ranges from 9 to 22 days, while the luteal phase ranges from 12 to 14 days. As a result, the normal menstrual cycle can vary from 21 to 36 days. Longer or shorter cycles are much more common at the extremes of reproductive age, a reflection of developing or deteriorating ovarian function.

Endometrial cycle

The endometrium undergoes cyclical regeneration and disintegration as a result of the influences of estrogen and progesterone (Figure 1.3). It is

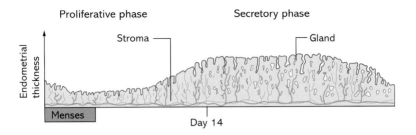

Figure 1.3 The endometrium undergoes regeneration and disintegrates during the menstrual cycle.

made up of glands supported on a stroma that contains fibroblasts and white blood cells. The cycle is divided into the proliferative phase, which is controlled by estrogen, and the secretory phase, which is controlled by progesterone. By the time of implantation the glands in the endometrium are coiled and twisted, and secrete many factors that are important for the support of a developing embryo. If no pregnancy occurs, the concentration of progesterone will drop. In response to this, the spiral arterioles that supply the endometrium will undergo vasospasm, which leads to necrosis and desquamation of the endometrium. This appears as menstruum and contains the sloughed endometrium, a large amount of mucus and a proportion of blood. Soon after menstruation the epithelium of the endometrium starts to regenerate and another cycle starts. Average menstrual loss is approximately 30 ml and the 95% confidence limit is 77 ml.

Control of menstruation

Clearly estrogen and progesterone are crucial in the normal development of the endometrium and the initiation of menstruation. Abnormalities in the absolute levels of these hormones or in their timing within the cycle may lead to abnormalities of endometrial growth, which may cause abnormal menstruation. The speed with which the spiral arterioles relax after the vasospasm may lead to heavy bleeding if other hemostatic mechanisms are not in place. This spasm of the arterioles appears to be under the control of prostaglandins in the endometrium. Abnormalities in local clotting mechanisms will alter menstrual flow, especially the action of fibrinolysis which, if excessive, may lead to breakdown of the clots that close the arterioles. Finally, the speed of regeneration of the endometrial epithelium will alter menstrual loss, as this regeneration is an important hemostatic mechanism.

Key references

Berek JS. *Novak's Gynecology.* 12th edn. Baltimore: Williams & Wilkins, 1996.

Shaw RW, Soutter P, Stanton S. *Gynaecology.* 2nd edn. Edinburgh: Churchill Livingstone, 1997.

Dysfunctional uterine bleeding (DUB) is defined as heavy regular menstrual bleeding for which no cause can be found on history, examination or investigation. The other main term used to describe this problem is menorrhagia but it is becoming more common to use DUB.

Epidemiology

The complaint of DUB is most common in women in their late 30s and 40s, though it can occur in teenagers within the first few years of menarche. One of the most interesting facets of this problem is the consistent finding, both in Europe and North America, that fewer than 50% of women attending a gynecological clinic complaining of heavy menstruation actually have the problem when the loss is objectively measured.

At any time, over 2 million women in the UK will be taking the oral contraceptive pill, resulting in decreased menstrual loss of up to 50%. Therefore, many women may have a lower menstrual loss than normal for many years but consider their normal loss to be heavy when they stop taking the oral contraceptive. It is also naive to consider that it is the loss alone about which women are complaining. It is very likely that it is a combination of the blood loss, the social inconvenience, dysmenorrhea and the premenstrual syndrome (PMS) that constitutes DUB. These considerations are very important when considering the management of the problem.

Pathogenesis

Although DUB is most common at extremes of reproductive age, there is no evidence that women with objectively heavy periods have abnormal endocrinology in their menstrual cycles compared with those with normal loss. There is good evidence of abnormalities in endometrial prostaglandin metabolism and in local coagulation mechanisms in women with heavy periods. The reasons why these occur are unknown. Whether fibroids cause DUB is debated and this will be discussed later. Heavy periods were thought to be common after female sterilization, but there is a comparable increase in the complaint in the spouses of men who have had a vasectomy, suggesting that the problem is one of perception of the loss. Thyroid disease and systemic coagulation disorders (either primary or secondary to drug therapy) can cause heavy periods, but these causes must be considered rare.

History

A full gynecological history should be taken; the aspects that are of particular importance are shown in Table 2.1.

Examination

A detailed abdominal and pelvic examination must be performed. Of particular importance are:
• the finding of an abdominal mass
• the appearance of the cervix
• the size and position of the uterus
• adnexal tenderness or masses.

TABLE 2.1

Patient history required for investigation of DUB

- Cycle length
- Length of menstruation
- Passage of clots and flooding
- Number of tampons and towels used during a period
- Any intermenstrual or postcoital bleeding
- Flooding of bed at night
- Menopausal symptoms
- Recent contraception
- Recent male or female sterilization
- Dysmenorrhea
- Premenstrual syndrome

Investigations

The investigations that may be conducted are outlined in Table 2.2.

Plan of management

A simple algorithm for the management of DUB in general practice is shown in Figure 2.1, based on the premise that the woman has a normal history, examination and smear. Referral to a gynecologist is generally unnecessary unless there are abnormalities in any of these parameters.

Investigations by the gynecologist

The main investigations initiated by a gynecologist are pelvic ultrasound scan and hysteroscopy.

Ultrasound scans are indicated if the clinician considers there to be abnormalities on examination or if an adequate examination is not possible due to lack of patient cooperation and/or obesity.

Hysteroscopy (Figure 2.2) has replaced dilatation and curettage as the investigation of choice for menstrual disturbance. It can be performed on an outpatient basis without a general anesthetic. It enables complete visualization of the uterine cavity and diagnosis of endometrial polyps and submucous fibroids that may have been missed by other techniques. Hysteroscopy may be indicated in women under 45 years with increased

TABLE 2.2

Investigations conducted for DUB

Smear	Essential unless there is objective evidence of normality within past 3 years
Hemoglobin	Essential; anemia will support the history but a normal hemoglobin level does not rule out DUB
Coagulation studies	Only if there is a history to suggest a disorder
Thyroid function	Only if there is a suspicion of thyroid disorder in history or on examination

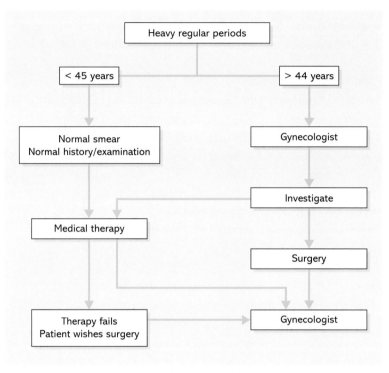

Figure 2.1 Management of dysfunctional uterine bleeding.

risk of endometrial carcinoma, e.g. with obesity, or with intermenstrual
bleeding.

Medical treatment

There are three main medical treatment options for DUB: non-steroidal
anti-inflammatory drugs (NSAIDs), fibrinolytic inhibitors and
exogenous synthetic reproductive steroids.

NSAIDs work by changing the amounts of prostaglandins in the
endometrium. Considerable evidence exists to show that they will
decrease menstrual blood loss by approximately 20%, especially in
women with proven heavy loss. NSAIDs are also effective in the
treatment of dysmenorrhea. Because they are only used during
menstruation, NSAIDs have limited side-effects and can usually be used
in the long term.

(a)

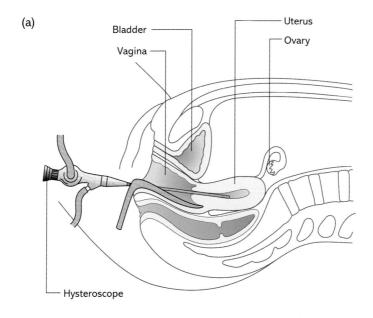

(b)

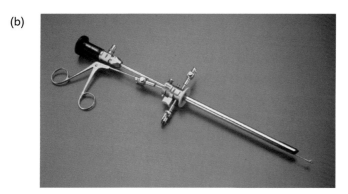

Figure 2.2 In hysteroscopy (a), the hysteroscope (b) is passed into the vagina and through the cervix in order to examine the endometrium and sample or remove polyps from the endometrial cavity under direct vision.

Fibrinolytic inhibitors, such as tranexamic acid, work by stopping fibrinolysis of the clots in the spiral arterioles, thus increasing hemostasis. They are undoubtedly effective and have been reported to decrease blood loss by around 40%. Again, their efficacy is greatest in those patients with proven heavy loss. Although there may be anxiety

17

about associated systemic thrombotic complications, large population studies in Scandinavia have failed to show this. Fibrinolytic inhibitors need only be taken during menstruation; they have a limited number of minor side-effects and can therefore be used in the long term. It should be noted that these medications are not licensed in the USA.

Synthetic steroids. There are three ways in which synthetic steroids can be used to treat DUB:
- to impose a menstrual cycle
- to compensate for abnormal endogenous endocrine secretion
- to suppress the menstrual cycle completely.

Imposition of a menstrual cycle. The most effective agent for this is the oral contraceptive. It is simple, has a limited number of side-effects and will decrease menstrual loss by an average of 30%. In individuals with no risk factors, it can be used over the age of 40 and has the added benefit of treating dysmenorrhea in many women. It is particularly useful in teenagers. For these reasons the oral contraceptive should be considered as first-line treatment for menstrual disorders.

Compensation for abnormal secretion. For over 30 years it has been common practice to prescribe synthetic progestogens in the luteal phase of the menstrual cycle (days 15–25). The logic for this rests on the premise that the luteal phase is endocrinologically abnormal in women with regular heavy periods although, as stated previously, there is no evidence to support this hypothesis. More importantly, there is little evidence that the prescription of progestogens in the luteal phase decreases menstrual blood loss and, until consistent data exist, this treatment has little to recommend it.

Suppression of the menstrual cycle. The aim of these treatments is to create amenorrhea. Continuous synthetic progestogens are effective and are well tolerated by some women. Problems with fluid retention and poor bleeding control may exist in others. Danazol is a synthetic androgen, and a large body of data exists on its efficacy in precipitating amenorrhea and decreasing menstrual loss. However, androgenic side-effects can lead to poor tolerability in up to 20% of patients, and long-term use can lead to liver dysfunction, so liver function should be monitored after 6 months' treatment. It is nevertheless a very effective therapy, particularly in the short term. GnRH agonists will successfully precipitate amenorrhea, but are associated with menopausal side-effects: the hypo-estrogenic state results in bone demineralization. As a result, these drugs can only be used for up to 6 months.

The Mirena intrauterine system. While conventional intrauterine devices (IUDs) are associated with increased menstrual loss, the Mirena intrauterine system releases levonorgestrel into the endometrium continuously, resulting in reduced menstrual loss and dysmenorrhea, and often amenorrhea. The device is now licensed for this indication in the UK. Women need to be informed that up to 6 months' use is required before the device is fully effective.

Failure of medical therapy. Every practitioner will be aware of the poor efficacy of medical therapy in DUB. Probably the main reason for this is that at least 50% of DUB patients do not have an objectively heavy loss and the majority of drugs are most efficacious in those with objectively heavy loss. Only those drugs that precipitate amenorrhea will succeed in women with a normal loss, but unfortunately their side-effects and expense mean that they do not represent a logical alternative for long-term therapy. It is therefore inevitable that many patients opt for a surgical solution after they have experienced failure of medical therapy.

Surgical therapy

Currently there are two main surgical approaches to the problem of DUB: hysterectomy or endometrial ablation.

Hysterectomy. Classically, either vaginal or abdominal hysterectomy has been the mainstay of surgical treatment of menstrual disorders (Figure 2.3). Recently there has been some feeling that hysterectomy represents an excessive way of dealing with these problems and is used uncritically by gynecologists. To counter this, it needs to be reiterated that the operation virtually guarantees a cure of DUB and that studies of patients after hysterectomy have all reported a high level of satisfaction

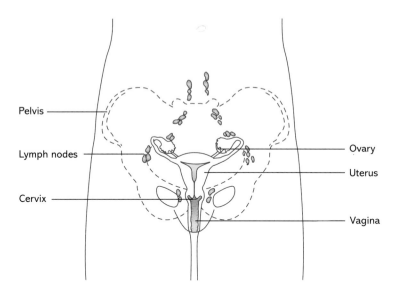

Pelvis

Lymph nodes

Cervix

Ovary

Uterus

Vagina

Figure 2.3 In a total hysterectomy, the uterus and cervix are removed. In a subtotal hysterectomy, only the uterus is removed.

with the operation; the most common complaint was the length of time it took for their medical practitioner to recommend it!

Although there are risks associated with hysterectomy, these must be considered slight in a fit woman below the age of 50. A small number of women do, however, experience psychosexual problems following hysterectomy. Because of the benefits provided, hysterectomy must be considered the benchmark against which all other treatments of DUB, either medical or surgical, are judged.

Surgical practice is increasingly oriented towards vaginal rather than abdominal hysterectomy because of the shorter recovery time and reduced operative morbidity. Laparoscopic procedures such as laparoscopic supracervical hysterectomy are becoming established in US practice, though the long-term outcomes of laparoscopic procedures remain to be established.

Endometrial ablation has become established as a satisfactory alternative to hysterectomy. The uterus is left behind, and these operations can be performed as day cases. Clearly, these techniques are appealing to clinicians, patients and health managers, but care is needed in patient selection as they are not effective in treating dysmenorrhea. A variety of well-established methods are available for destruction of the endometrium (Figure 2.4). Other available modalities include thermal balloon ablation and microwave endometrial ablation. Long-term follow-up studies will clarify which of the available techniques gives the best results.

Overall, approximately 75% of women are satisfied with the results of endometrial ablation and do not require further surgery, whereas the remaining 25% are likely to proceed to hysterectomy. There is an advantage to be gained by the preoperative thinning of the endometrium using danazol or, more conveniently, a single dose of a long-acting GnRH agonist such as goserelin. This results in a technically easier procedure and may lead to more reliable destruction of the basal layer of the endometrium.

(a)

(b)

(c)

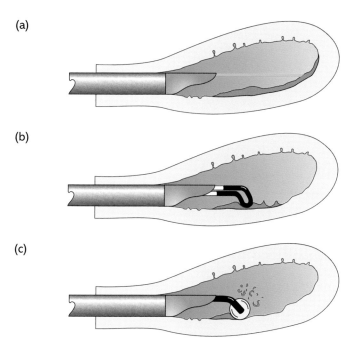

Figure 2.4 Endometrial ablation may be performed with (a) a laser, (b) a wire loop, or (c) a revolving ball.

Key reference

RCOG Guidelines Series.
*Management of Menorrhagia in
Secondary Care.*
www.rcog.org.uk/guidelines.asp?Page
ID=108&GuidelineID=29

The three most usual forms of abnormal vaginal bleeding are intermenstrual, postcoital and postmenopausal. They often have a common etiology and involve similar investigations and management.

Definitions

Intermenstrual bleeding is defined as any bleeding occurring within a regular menstrual cycle but not at menstruation. Postcoital bleeding is any bleeding occurring after sexual intercourse. Both are common phenomena, frequently occur intermittently and rarely signal major pathology in the premenopausal woman. Occasionally, however, they are symptoms of potentially fatal disease and it is important that the clinician has a clear plan for their management. Postmenopausal bleeding is defined as an episode of vaginal bleeding occurring more than 1 year after the presumed menopause; it may or may not be related to intercourse.

Pathogenesis

Common causes for abnormal bleeding are usually local to the vagina and cervix (Table 3.1). Most of these causes are self-evident and do not need further explanation to a qualified doctor. However, the three most common – physiological, cervical ectropion and the oral contraceptive – can cause some confusion and will be described in more detail.

Physiological. The fluctuations in the serum concentrations of estrogen during a normal menstrual cycle have been discussed in Chapter 1. A large rise occurs during the follicular phase, followed by a precipitate fall for 2 to 3 days at the time of ovulation. In some women, this fall can be so large that the endometrium loses its hormonal support in the same way as at menstruation. Desquamation commences but stops when estrogen and progesterone from the corpus luteum stimulate the endometrium. For this reason, consistent mid-cycle intermenstrual bleeding is a normal phenomenon in a young woman.

TABLE 3.1

Common causes of abnormal bleeding

Postmenopausal

- Atrophic vaginitis
- Cervical carcinoma
- Carcinoma of the endometrium

Intermenstrual and postcoital

- Physiological
- Cervical ectropion
- Oral contraceptive
- Vulvitis
- Cervical carcinoma

Cervical ectropion. The cervix is composed of two types of epithelium: columnar and squamous. The columnar epithelium is usually inside the cervical canal and is not visible, whereas the squamous epithelium covers the intra-vaginal portion of the cervix and is visible (Figure 3.1). The area where the two epithelia meet is called the squamo-columnar junction (S-CJ). The epithelia can change from one form to another under various conditions and therefore the S-CJ can move up or down the cervix. Movement of the S-CJ typically happens at times of high estrogen exposure such as puberty, during oral contraceptive use and during pregnancy. An ectropion occurs when the S-CJ moves down the cervix (Figure 3.1).

The columnar epithelium is translucent and blood vessels are visible to an observer. The squamous epithelium is opaque and appears dull. If the columnar epithelium becomes visible, it appears as a reddened area – the so-called ectropion. However, this is a misnomer and the appearances are physiological. The main problems caused by the columnar epithelium becoming intravaginal are that it can alter the vaginal discharge or, because the epithelium is fragile, it can be traumatized during intercourse and bleed. Unless either of these symptoms is considered a problem, there is no need to treat an ectropion as long as the smear is normal.

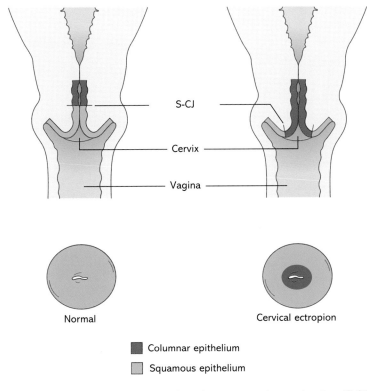

Figure 3.1 Cervical ectropion occurs when the squamo-columnar junction (S-CJ) moves down the cervix. The columnar epithelium appears as a reddened area, known as the ectropion.

Oral contraceptive. Doses of synthetic estrogen and progestogen in the oral contraceptive maintain the integrity of the endometrium during the 3 weeks that the pill is taken. There may be pharmacodynamic reasons why some women do not absorb a particular estrogen or progestogen efficiently, or the endometrium may not respond well to those compounds. If this is the case, there will be endometrial shedding and the woman will report intermenstrual bleeding. This is very common in the first few months of starting a new pill. If it is persistent, the doctor should prescribe a pill with differing doses of estrogen and progestogen. If the examination and smear are normal, there is virtually no chance that the bleeding heralds any serious pathology.

Investigation by the family physician

Obviously a complete history and examination are vital, and if infection is suspected, high vaginal and intracervical bacteriological swabs should be taken. A cervical smear should also be taken if needed.

Management

Postmenopausal bleeding. All cases of postmenopausal bleeding should be referred to a gynecologist.

Intermenstrual and postcoital bleeding. An algorithm for the management of these disorders is shown in Figure 3.2. Although many

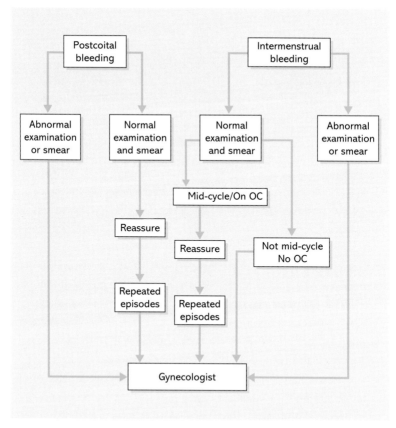

Figure 3.2 Management of intermenstrual and postcoital bleeding. OC, oral contraceptive.

of the avenues end with referral to a gynecologist, the majority of patients will have a normal examination and smear and will experience only one or two episodes of mid-cycle bleeding or be taking the oral contraceptive. Consequently, referral is not usually required.

Further investigation by the gynecologist

If the smear is abnormal, the gynecologist will institute colposcopy and cervical biopsy. The most important information required by the gynecologist in each of these disorders is whether the examination and smear are normal and whether there are any abnormalities in the endometrium. Traditionally this was determined by a D & C, but developments in ultrasound imaging, outpatient endometrial biopsy and hysteroscopy mean that the D & C has been superseded.

Treatment

The treatment of gynecological malignancy is outside the remit of this book. Vulvitis and atrophic vaginitis are treated by the application of the appropriate antifungal or hormonal agents. If a cervical ectropion continues to cause intermenstrual bleeding, it may be necessary to treat it in order to decrease symptoms. Commonly the columnar epithelium is destroyed by either cryocautery or diathermy and the squamous epithelium regrows over the location of the ectropion. This cannot be guaranteed, however, and if the cause of the ectropion, for example the continued use of the oral contraceptive, continues then it is likely that the ectropion will return.

Key references

Alexopoulos ED, Fay TN, Simonis CD. A review of 2581 out-patient diagnostic hysteroscopies in the management of abnormal uterine bleeding. *Gynaecol Endosc* 1999;8: 105–110.

Rosenthal AN, Panoskaltsis T, Smith T, Soutter WP. The frequency of significant pathology in women attending a general gynaecological service for postcoital bleeding. *Br J Obstet Gynaecol* 2001:108:103–106.

Disorders of ovulation

Ovulation resulting from the LH surge is one of the most important events in reproduction and determines the length of the menstrual cycle. Disorders of ovulation will present in two ways: absence or irregularity of the cycle and infertility.

Causes of ovulatory disorders

The simplest way to remember the main causes of ovulatory disorders is to work from the brain downwards to the ovary. The causes can then be divided into cerebral, hypothalamic–pituitary, thyroid, adrenal, ovarian and uterine/vaginal (Figure 4.1). Endometrial disorders can cause amenorrhea, although they are not strictly related to abnormal ovulation.

Cerebral. It is well recognized that vigorous exercise and stress, for example before academic examinations, will cause amenorrhea. Anorexia nervosa is typified by amenorrhea, but this occurs before the degree of weight loss is such that it could be fully explained nutritionally. Certain psychotropic medications will also cause disruption of the menstrual cycle. The mechanism of action of the above is presumed to be through alterations of the neurotransmitters that control the hypothalamus.

Hypothalamic–pituitary. Rare congenital disorders of the hypothalamus exist, such as Kallmann's syndrome. The most common pituitary causes of ovulatory disorders are neoplastic, in particular prolactinoma. Such conditions cause dysfunction of the pituitary either because of their local effects or as a result of their treatment by surgery or radiotherapy. A prolactinoma may present with galactorrhea and any pituitary tumor may present with visual disturbances. Finally, severe blood loss can lead to acute ischemic necrosis of the pituitary – Sheehan's syndrome. Classically this occurred after postpartum hemorrhage although this is rare nowadays in developed countries.

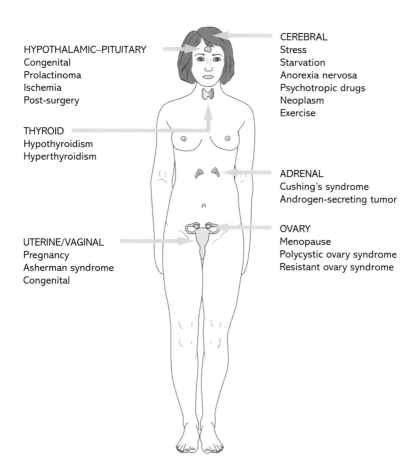

Figure 4.1 Causes of ovulatory disorders.

Thyroid disease. Either hypo- or hyperthyroidism can cause disorders of ovulation, although it is very rare for this to be the only presentation of the disease.

Adrenal disease. Amenorrhea can be a symptom in Cushing's syndrome. There are also rare androgen-secreting tumors of the adrenal that will cause suppression of the menstrual cycle as well as other symptoms of androgenization.

Ovarian disease is the most common and least understood reason for disorders of ovulation. Obviously the menopause occurring at an early age is one possible cause. The menopause is associated with an absence of ovarian follicles. Occasionally ovarian failure may occur while there are still many follicles, the so-called resistant ovary syndrome, which is thought to have an immunological basis. However, the most frequent problem is that the ovary fails to respond to LH and FSH in a coordinated and synchronous fashion. The reasons for this are unknown, but are thought to involve local factors through which one cell controls the behavior of its neighbors, i.e. paracrine control. Ovulation disorders based in the ovaries will have some aspects of polycystic ovary syndrome (PCOS). It is also possible to have ovarian dysfunction as a result of external factors, such as obesity, and there will be aspects of this that occur in PCOS.

Uterine/vaginal. The most common cause of amenorrhea in a fertile female is pregnancy and this must always be checked despite protestations to the contrary! Vigorous curettage can remove the endometrium completely, causing menstruation to cease – a condition known as Asherman syndrome. Certain congenital defects, such as absence of the endometrium or vagina, or an imperforate hymen, can present as amenorrhea.

Polycystic ovary syndrome

PCOS is a very common diagnosis that warrants a separate heading. Classically, PCOS presents with obesity, hirsutism, oligomenorrhea and infertility. The ovaries are enlarged with thickened stroma and there are

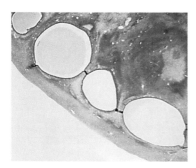

Figure 4.2 Histological appearance of a polycystic ovary. Note peripherally distributed follicles. Image courtesy of Dr Nita Singh.

many small cysts of approximately 7 mm diameter, situated peripherally under a thickened capsule (Figure 4.2). Endocrine investigations show raised concentrations of androgens and abnormalities in the concentrations of LH and FSH, with the former being raised. Ultrasonography shows that the classic description is at one end of a spectrum and that many women have only one or a few of the presenting features. For example, the ultrasound appearance of polycystic ovaries may occur in normal fertile women with no symptoms.

The cause of PCOS is unknown and it is likely that the final appearance of the ovary can occur as a result of a number of mechanisms. It is common to describe this as a self-perpetuating

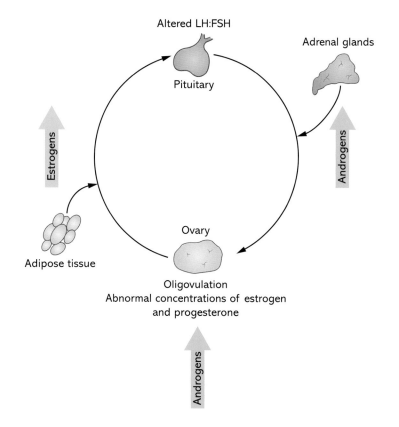

Figure 4.3 The self-perpetuating cycle of polycystic ovary syndrome.

circle, as shown in Figure 4.3. The syndrome may result from abnormalities anywhere within the circle, but the most common reasons are primary ovarian dysfunction or obesity. Androgens are converted to estrogens in peripheral adipose tissue and this is the main source of estrogens after the menopause. Premenopausal obese women will have high levels of estrogens which are thought to disturb the feedback control to the pituitary and thus initiate the problem. Women with PCOS are also insulin resistant, although whether this is a primary or a secondary phenomenon is unknown.

Currently, it is considered that the finding of polycystic ovaries on ultrasonography is the main diagnostic criterion (Figure 4.4). The endocrine findings typically reflect the clinical presentation. For example, LH levels are elevated in those with cycle disturbance, and free testosterone is elevated in those with hirsutism. However, it is possible to have some of the endocrine problems without the classic ultrasound findings.

Investigation of ovulatory disorders

A thorough patient history is vital. It is important to determine whether the problem is amenorrhea or oligomenorrhea; primary amenorrhea is defined as the absence of menstruation after 18 years of age. The time of onset and association with any symptoms suggestive of an intracranial tumor should be investigated. The occurrence of stressful

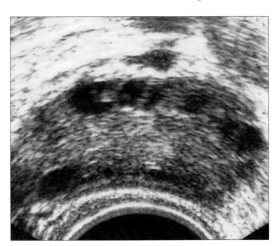

Figure 4.4 Classically, polycystic ovaries present as small, numerous peripheral cysts on ultrasound. Image courtesy of Dr Alex Lawrence.

events, psychological problems and changes in weight or exercise regime are important. Specific questions about galactorrhea should be asked. On examination, the height:weight ratio should be determined to check for obesity. Signs of androgenization such as hirsutism, clitoromegaly and hoarse voice should be searched for. It is also important to perform a vaginal examination.

Figure 4.5 is an algorithm for the investigation of ovulatory disorders. Individual practitioners should decide how much of the investigation they wish to perform. However, it is generally accepted

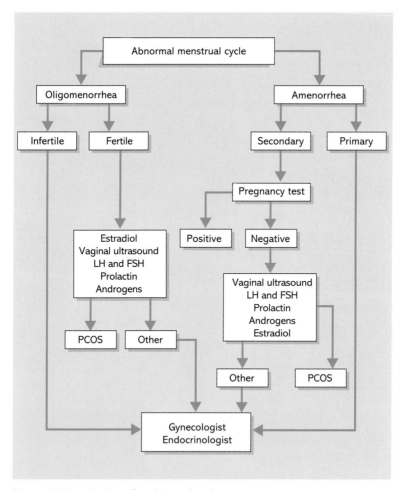

Figure 4.5 Investigation of ovulatory disorders.

that early referral to a specialist should occur to ensure that no serious, albeit rare, conditions such as brain, pituitary, adrenal or ovarian neoplasm are present.

Management of ovulatory disorders

Amenorrhea. The main management principle for amenorrhea is diagnostic. Having established an accurate diagnosis, the correct treatment strategy can then be initiated. Primary amenorrhea is usually just delayed puberty. If the problem is congenital hypothalamic disease, then the patient will need replacement therapy for pituitary hormones. Outflow obstruction in the vagina will require surgical treatment by a gynecologist. Hormone replacement therapy is used in cases of secondary amenorrhea due to premature menopause. Cerebral or pituitary tumors should be treated with surgery or radiotherapy. Prolactinomas can be treated medically with bromocriptine.

Oligomenorrhea

Infertility. If a woman is complaining of infertility both she and her partner will require a full investigation to establish a normal semen analysis and patent tubes before an ovulatory disorder is accepted as the cause. There are two main therapies for induction of ovulation: anti-estrogens and exogenous gonadotropins.

Anti-estrogens. The typical drug used for this is clomiphene, a potent anti-estrogen which blocks the estrogen feedback to the pituitary. This leads to an increase in LH and FSH, which in turn stimulates follicular growth. Clomiphene is administered from day 2 to day 6 of the menstrual cycle at a daily dose of 50–200 mg. A certain level of endogenous estrogen should be present in order that the signal may be blocked; a functioning pituitary secreting LH and FSH is also required. Patients should be advised of a small but significant risk of multiple pregnancy. The duration of treatment should only exceptionally exceed 6 months.

Exogenous gonadotropins. If there are low concentrations of endogenous estrogen or if the pituitary is not functioning, then the treatment is to give gonadotropins by injection. Menotropin contains 75 IU of LH and 75 IU of FSH. It should only be used by trained practitioners as it is very easy to hyperstimulate the ovary and to cause multiple pregnancies. Careful monitoring of follicular growth, by ultrasound, and of plasma estradiol concentration is essential. Newer preparations now use genetically produced LH and FSH in several different ratios. These preparations should be used only under specialist supervision.

Irregular cycles. There is no clear necessity to treat irregular cycles alone. It is valid simply to inform the patient of any diagnosis of PCOS and explain its main implications. General advice about weight loss, where applicable, should be given. The oral contraceptive can be used to provide a regular cycle. This has the added benefit of increasing the concentration of sex-hormone-binding globulin in serum, which may diminish the androgenic manifestations of the syndrome. Patients should be advised that they may require ovulation induction to become pregnant, but should be reassured that the oral contraceptive will not increase the need for it. They should also be advised that there is evidence that women with PCOS may have a higher miscarriage rate.

Key reference

Mason H. Polycystic ovary syndrome. In: Stones RW (ed) *Gynaecology Highlights 2000–01*. Oxford: Health Press, 2001.

Pelvic pain is defined as a subjective complaint of pain in the lower abdomen or pelvis which may be either acute or chronic, constant or cyclical, and spontaneous or precipitated by intercourse. It is the second most common reason for a woman to be referred to a gynecologist.

Causes of pelvic pain

Table 5.1 describes the common causes of pelvic pain. There are many rare causes, but the ones described here cover most diagnoses for patients seen in routine practice.

Previous sexual abuse. There is a significant association between sexual victimization before the age of 15 years and later chronic pelvic pain. The care provider should always question the patient in this regard.

General investigation

A detailed history is vital. The onset, timing and quality of the pain should be determined, as well as any relationship to the menstrual cycle. A number of relevant questions should also be asked. If dyspareunia occurs, is it superficial or deep and does it happen every time? Are there any precipitating or relieving factors? Is there any history of pelvic infection, a previous ectopic pregnancy or pelvic surgery? Are there any associated bowel or urinary symptoms? It is important to make a positive diagnosis of psychological disturbance by enquiring about prime symptoms of anxiety or depression.

A thorough pelvic examination should be carried out. An entirely normal vaginal examination makes the diagnosis of gynecological causes much less likely. Rectal examination is also important as it complements vaginal examination and gives access to the posterior compartment of the pelvis.

Algorithms for the investigation and management of acute and chronic pelvic pain are shown in Figures 5.1 and 5.2, respectively. All patients with their first episode of acute pelvic pain should be admitted

TABLE 5.1

Common causes of pelvic pain

Acute

Gynecological	Non-gynecological
• Infection	• Cystitis
• Endometriosis	• Appendicitis
• Ectopic pregnancy	• Colitis
• Cyst accident (torsion or bleeding)	
• Torsion of a fibroid	
• Dysmenorrhea	

Chronic

Gynecological	Non-gynecological
• Pelvic inflammatory disease	• Irritable bowel disease
• Endometriosis	• Musculo-skeletal
• Adhesions	• Bowel–urinary neoplasm
• Fibroids	• Neuropathic
• Ovarian cyst	
• Venous congestion	

to hospital. Even if the diagnosis appears to be obvious, as in acute pelvic inflammatory disease, it is important that it is verified. The most important aspect of the investigation of chronic pelvic pain is a good history and examination. From these the practitioner can determine which is the likely system involved and which investigations should be conducted; many of these can be carried out by the family physician.

The need for and timing of laparoscopy are very much dependent upon individual clinicians. It is a safe investigation and whether or not there is a positive or negative diagnosis, it provides important information.

Management of acute pelvic pain

Ectopic pregnancy. Classically, ectopic pregnancy presents as acute-onset, severe lower abdominal pain in a woman with amenorrhea and

symptoms of pregnancy. It is more common in women:
- taking the progesterone-only oral contraceptive
- with an IUD in situ
- with a past history of tubal surgery.

Typically, there are signs of abdominal and pelvic peritonitis. However, ectopic pregnancy can present as slow-onset pain with a history of abnormal menstrual bleeding, either in timing or quality. Referral to a specialist is vital if ectopic pregnancy is suspected. Treatment options include expectant management, methotrexate, laparoscopic surgery or, in extreme cases where the patient is collapsed, urgent laparotomy and salpingectomy.

Pelvic infection. There is strong argument for a laparoscopy during the initial acute episode in order to verify the diagnosis and obtain

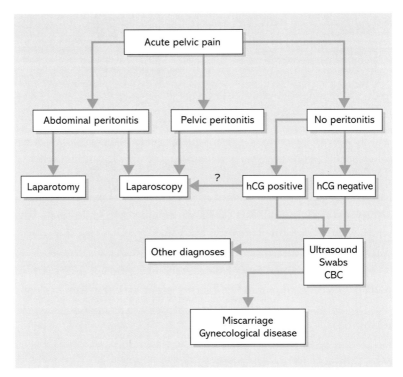

Figure 5.1 Investigation and management of acute pelvic pain. hCG, human chorionic gonadotropin; CBC, complete blood cell count (FBC in the UK).

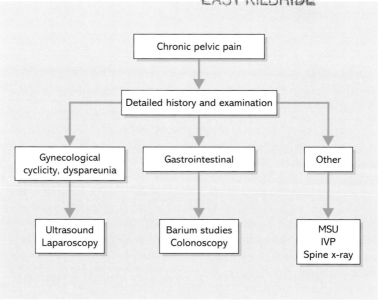

Figure 5.2 Investigation and management of chronic pelvic pain. MSU, mid-stream urine; IVP, intravenous pyelography.

bacteriological swabs from the fimbrial ends of the fallopian tubes. Intravenous or oral antibiotics should be prescribed; the route of administration will depend on the clinical condition of the patient. Tracing of previous sexual partners by genitourinary physicians is an important part of management.

Ovarian cyst. Conservative management is appropriate if the pain is moderate and there are few physical signs. If this is not the case, a laparoscopy or laparotomy should be performed.

Miscarriage. There is no active treatment for a threatened miscarriage. Ultrasonography can determine whether there is a viable fetus. If there is not, then evacuation of the uterus can be performed and the woman does not have to face many days of uncertainty. If there is a viable fetus, she can be reassured that the pregnancy is likely to continue. This investigation can be performed by the family physician, but heavy bleeding will require hospitalization.

Management of chronic pelvic pain

Endometriosis. The management of this is described in Chapter 6.

Pelvic inflammatory disease is a common diagnosis for chronic pelvic pain and usually the one with the least objective support. It is essential that there is laparoscopic verification of the diagnosis. Clinicians should beware the patient with this diagnosis who appears not to improve in spite of repeated courses of antibiotics – it may be that the diagnosis is wrong rather than the treatment. If the diagnosis is verified, long-term antibiotics can help, but often the final solution is a pelvic clearance.

Ovarian cyst/fibroid. The management of symptomatic ovarian cysts is usually surgical; management of fibroids is discussed in Chapter 7.

Irritable bowel syndrome is a very common cause of pelvic pain and is estimated to be the diagnosis in up to 50% of presentations. Care should be taken with history and the presence of abdominal distension at times other than menstruation; abdominal pain more than once a month and a disordered bowel habit should be specifically queried. The management of this problem is outside the remit of this book. The interested reader may like to refer to *Irritable Bowel Syndrome* in the *Fast Facts* series.

Psychological problems are common in pelvic pain, but most often occur as a result of the chronic problem. Diagnosis is not just one of exclusion; it is important to ensure that an organic disease is not present, but it is also necessary to look for positive symptoms of psychological dysfunction. Examples of this would be recent life events, mood disturbances and sleep disorders.

It is essential to establish the patient's own priorities, for example if she wishes to pursue a definitive diagnosis for her pain. There has been interest in conscious pain mapping by laparoscopy in women with chronic pelvic pain. The procedure is especially useful to establish the relevance of potentially coincidental findings such as the presence of adhesions. Alternatively, the patient may prefer to focus on symptomatic treatment with GnRH analogs or progestogens.

Key references

Carter JF. Nongynecologic causes of chronic pelvic pain. *The Female Patient* 2000;25:33–43.

Howard FM, El-Minawi AM, Sanchez RA. Conscious pain mapping by laparoscopy in women with chronic pelvic pain. *Obstet Gynecol* 2000;96:934–9.

Lampe A, Sölder E, Ennemoser A et al. Chronic pelvic pain and previous sexual abuse. *Obstet Gynecol* 2000;96:929–32.

Endometriosis is defined as the presence of tissue histologically similar to endometrium outside the uterine cavity and the myometrium. It is most commonly found in the pelvis, but may also be present in the abdominal cavity, the pleura and, very rarely, in limbs and the brain.

Etiology and pathogenesis

The main etiological factors that control the appearance of endometriosis are shown in Table 6.1. Clearly, factors that increase the exposure to menstruation increase the likelihood of the disease occurring, whereas those that decrease the exposure protect against it. It can be concluded that menstruation is an important factor in the pathogenesis of endometriosis. As modern woman is experiencing more menstruation than previously, this would explain why there appears to be an increased incidence of the disease.

Menstruum not only flows down the vagina but also refluxes along the fallopian tubes and into the pelvis. It is this refluxed menstruum that is thought to be the cause of endometriosis. How menstruum actually causes the disease has not been proven, and the main theories of pathogenesis are described in the following sections.

Implantation. Menstruum that refluxes along the fallopian tubes is viable. It implants on the ovaries and peritoneum and

TABLE 6.1

Etiology of endometriosis

• Age	• Frequent cycles
• Family history	• Nulliparity
• Heavy periods	• No history of contraceptive use

subsequently responds to ovarian hormone. Currently, this is thought to be the most likely pathogenesis for the occurrence of the disease in the pelvis.

Celomic metaplasia. The peritoneal epithelium in the pelvis can change from a simple form into endometrial epithelium (metaplasia) in response to ovarian steroids.

Induction. The peritoneum metaplases to endometrium under the influence of factors released by the refluxed menstruum.

Mechanical transplantation. If endometrium is transplanted to a different location, e.g. on a surgical blade, it will implant. There is no doubt that mechanical transplantation occurs and this is shown by appearance of endometriosis in abdominal scars following operation on the uterus.

Vascular/lymphatic spread. Endometrium has been found in the blood vessels and lymph channels draining the uterus. This means of spread is thought to explain the appearance of disease in locations distant from the pelvis.

Visual presentation

Classically endometriosis is described as blue-black or 'powder burn' spots on the peritoneum, fallopian tubes and ovaries. Endometrial tissue has also been found in vesicular, clear, hemorrhagic and petechial lesions (Figure 6.1) and in white plaques, fibrous scars and even in normal peritoneum. In the ovaries, endometrial tissue can form large cysts containing a thick brown fluid – so-called 'chocolate' cysts. This fluid contains hemosiderin and is thought to result from bleeding inside the cyst. It can occur from bleeding in any cyst but is usually only very brown and thick in endometriosis.

From the above it will become clear that endometriosis is a much more common and variable disease than was previously thought. This important fact will be discussed later as it affects the management of the problem.

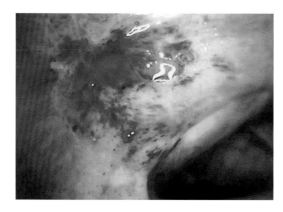

Figure 6.1
Hemorrhagic lesions on left uterosacral ligament.

Clinical presentation

Specific symptoms and signs are associated with endometriosis (Table 6.2). Cyclicity of pelvic pain and dyspareunia are classic symptoms, the latter being a particularly important problem for any woman in a relationship. Consequently, it should always be taken seriously and investigated. Tender nodules on the uterosacral ligaments are virtually pathognomonic of endometriosis. Other signs are not specific to endometriosis (Table 6.2).

It is important to stress that the appearance of endometriosis does not necessarily mean that it is the cause of the patient's symptoms. The

TABLE 6.2

Symptoms and signs of endometriosis

Symptoms
- Pelvic pain
- Dyspareunia
- Dysmenorrhea

Signs
- Tender nodules on the uterosacral ligaments
- Pelvic mass
- Fixed pelvis
- Pelvic tenderness

finding of endometriosis is common and will be coincidental with other disorders in some patients. The visual finding of the disease should, therefore, be accompanied by a recognizable symptom complex or physical signs before causality with the symptoms is accepted. This is probably the most contentious area in endometriosis at the moment.

Diagnosis

Although clinical history and signs may strongly suggest endometriosis, correct diagnosis can only be confirmed by visualization of the disease at laparoscopy. This means that referral to a gynecologist is essential and treatment should not be started without a formal diagnosis. This is particularly important as other diseases, such as ovarian neoplasm and pelvic inflammatory disease, can be difficult to distinguish from endometriosis without laparoscopy. Ultrasound is not helpful in the diagnosis of endometriosis, and no discriminating serum markers have been described, though CA125 may be elevated.

Relationship with infertility

Endometriosis is found more commonly in infertile women, possibly because such women do not experience the protective effect of pregnancy. Initially it was thought that this relationship was causal and the endometriosis was treated. If the endometriosis damages the tubes and ovaries, there is no doubt that it causes infertility. However, there is no evidence that the presence of endometriosis in itself causes infertility and no objective evidence that its successful medical treatment will improve fertility when compared with no treatment. As such, there is no indication for medical treatment of endometriosis in infertile women. This is especially important as medical treatments act as contraceptives and can have side-effects. Recent data from a large multicenter study suggest that ablation of endometriosis at diagnostic laparoscopy for infertility can improve fertility.

Medical treatment

NSAIDs act as inhibitors of prostaglandin synthesis and are particularly useful for dysmenorrhea. They are very effective and have limited side-effects because they are given for a short time period.

Progestogens. The synthetic progestogens, medroxyprogesterone acetate, norethisterone and dydrogesterone are all licensed for the treatment of endometriosis. Their mechanism of action involves decidualization and subsequent necrosis. Progestogens are effective and provide relief in 70–80% of patients. They have predictable progestogenic side-effects (weight gain and vaginal spotting) and are poorly tolerated in some patients.

Danazol is a synthetic androgen derived from 19-nortestosterone. It is very effective in causing androgenic atrophy and will provide symptom relief in up to 90% of patients. Unfortunately it has androgenic side-effects (weight gain, acne and greasy skin), which are poorly tolerated by up to 20% of patients.

GnRH agonists. As analogs of GnRH, these drugs suppress LH and FSH secretion from the pituitary. As a result, the ovary ceases to function and there is no secretion of estrogen. The latter is essential for the continued proliferation of endometriosis, and without it the endometrium shrinks. These drugs are very effective, providing relief of symptoms in up to 90% of patients. They have predictable menopausal side-effects of hot flushes and vaginal dryness, but appear to be better tolerated than danazol. GnRH agonists available in the UK include: leuprorelin acetate; goserelin; nafarelin; and buserelin. These are presented either as nasal sprays or depot injections. The estrogen deficiency-related adverse effects of GnRH agonists can be prevented by the concomitant administration of 'add-back' estrogen replacement, for example using tibolone. Add-back therapy does not substantially reduce the effectiveness of GnRH agonists and renders a course of treatment much more acceptable to the patient.

GnRH antagonists are competitive inhibitors – antagonistic activity follows receptor binding and results in blockage of either the receptor message or neurotransmission. The initial flare of estrogen is avoided, but side-effects from the prompt hypo-estrogenic state may be significant. GnRH antagonists are not licensed for use in the UK or USA.

Surgical treatment

Laparotomy and laparoscopy are the two main surgical options and each has particular advantages. Traditionally, laparotomy has been the mainstay of surgery. It is best for major surgery and allows removal of the uterus, tubes and ovaries. It is also useful in reconstructive surgery to the tubes and ovaries. Laparoscopy is now being used increasingly. It has benefits in that it is much less invasive, can be performed on a day-case basis and can be repeated if necessary. In addition, the magnifying power of the laparoscope allows accurate diagnosis and treatment with either laser or diathermy to ablate the disease. Only a few surgeons can perform complex surgery through a laparoscope.

Guidelines for the treatment of endometriosis

Endometriosis can be treated either medically or surgically. An algorithm for the management of endometriosis is shown in Figure 6.2.

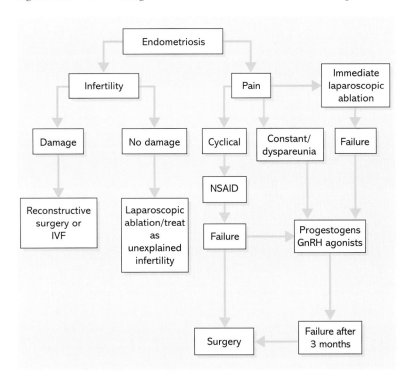

Figure 6.2 Management of endometriosis.

TABLE 6.3

Comparison of medical and surgical treatments for endometriosis

Medical	Surgical
• No damage to tubes and ovaries	• Can be performed at diagnosis
• Treatment can be repeated	• Reconstructive surgery possible
• Alternative therapies available	• More suitable for older women
• More suitable for younger women	• Useful if medical therapy fails
• Can be expensive	• No side-effects
• Side-effects	• Requires skilled surgeons
	• Equipment can be expensive
	• Cannot be done repeatedly

It is important to note that medical therapy should have an impact on symptoms within 3 months. If this has not occurred, the drug has failed and it should be replaced by one that uses a different mechanism. Broadly, the therapeutic impact and duration of benefit are proportional to the degree of ovarian suppression obtained and the duration of therapy; if the response is favorable, a 6-month course is conventional. The main agents in current use are progestogens and GnRH agonists. Danazol has largely been superseded because of androgenic adverse effects. The adverse effects of progestogens such as medroxyprogesterone acetate at a dose of 30 mg daily include weight gain and irregular bleeding. GnRH agonists will produce intense menopausal symptoms and result in reversible loss of bone mineral: these adverse effects can be prevented by the use of 'add-back' estrogen or estrogen/progestin combinations. An example of a suitable agent licensed for 'add-back' use in the UK is tibolone. The use of 'add-back' estrogen does not substantially diminish the efficacy of the GnRH agonist because ovarian suppression is maintained. GnRH agonists are more costly than progestogens, but with estrogen 'add-back' adverse effects are minimal.

It is important not to think of endometriosis as a curable disease. Clearly women continue to menstruate after medical or surgical treatment and therefore the mechanism that precipitates the disease persists. Studies have shown that there is a recurrence rate of 15–20% a year. If the disease returns within 6 months it is logical to consider that the treatment failed and to use another method or drug. If the gap is longer than 6 months then it is reasonable to conclude that the treatment worked but that the disease has returned; a repeat course of the same drug can therefore be given. Repeated failure of medical therapy determines that a surgical approach is better.

Medical and surgical approaches both have strengths and weaknesses (Table 6.3). In the final analysis, the best approach is individualized to each particular patient and is dependent on symptoms, the need to maintain fertility, the amount of the disease and previous treatments.

Key references

Hesla JS, Rock JA. Endometriosis. In: Rock JA, Thompson JD, eds. *TeLinde's Operative Gynecology.* 8th edn. Philadelphia, New York: Lippincott-Raven, 1997:585–624.

Prentice et al. Medical treatment of endometriosis-associated infertility. *Cochrane Library.* www.nelh.nhs.uk/cochrane.asp

Prior A, Whorwell PJ. Gynaecological consultation in patients with irritable bowel syndrome. *Gut* 1989;30:996–8.

Fibroids are leiomyomas (common benign tumors of the smooth muscle) of the myometrium (Figures 7.1 and 7.2).

Etiology and pathogenesis

The prevalence of fibroids is approximately 20% in the Caucasian population and up to 50% in Afro-Caribbeans and Afro-Americans. They are more common in first-order relatives of sufferers and less common in women of high parity. Fibroids are dependent upon estrogen for their growth and therefore are much more common in women of reproductive age. Molecular studies suggest they originate from one muscle cell (monoclonal). It is not known what initiates the abnormal growth, although there is evidence that local growth factors and/or cytogenetic aberrations play a role.

The natural history of fibroids is that shrinkage occurs after the menopause. There is a rare malignancy of uterine smooth muscle, a leiomyosarcoma, which is most common during the seventh decade.

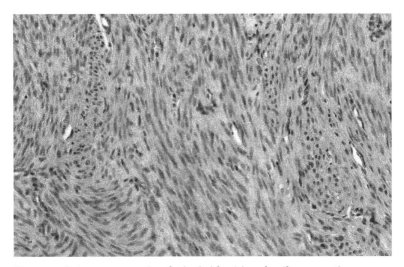

Figure 7.1 Leiomyomas consist of whorled fascicles of uniform smooth muscle cells.

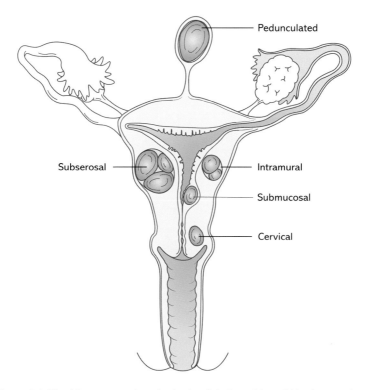

Figure 7.2 Fibroids are named on the basis of their position within the muscle.

The low incidence of the tumor, the considerable differential in the age of maximal incidence between it and fibroids, and cytogenetic evidence suggest that malignancy starts de novo and is not the result of a malignant change in a fibroid. There is therefore no imperative to remove an asymptomatic fibroid in order to avoid malignant change.

Complications

Fibroids do not cause problems in most women and are often undiagnosed. The problems that can result include:

- degeneration
- torsion
- calcification
- pelvic pressure symptoms
- abnormal uterine bleeding.

Degeneration is unusual and is either cystic or hyaline; a special type of necrosis called 'red degeneration' occurs only in pregnancy. If a fibroid is pedunculated it can become torted. Calcification is common but usually asymptomatic. Perhaps the most common symptoms that fibroids cause are feelings of pelvic pressure or discomfort. Occasionally they can press upon the bladder and cause frequency, difficulty with micturition or a feeling of incomplete emptying. Fibroids are often described as the cause of heavy menstruation. Good scientific evidence for this is absent and it is very difficult to see how a fibroid that does not abut the endometrial cavity can influence menstruation. It is possible that those that distort and enlarge the uterine cavity, the submucosal fibroids, may lead to a heavier loss especially if they increase the area of endometrium. However, this is also unproven.

Investigations

The most useful diagnostic tool for fibroids is pelvic ultrasound. This gives a clear picture of the fibroid, its size and position in the uterus; it is also possible to diagnose degeneration and malignant change. Full blood count is helpful as it can help to verify a diagnosis of DUB if there is anemia; in rare incidences fibroids will secrete erythropoietin, resulting in polycythemia. Computerized tomography (CT) scans or magnetic resonance imaging (MRI) can also be used to image fibroids, but these techniques are expensive and have little benefit above pelvic ultrasonography. Submucous fibroids, which may cause hypermenorrhea, can be visualized by hysteroscopy.

Clinical management

As previously stated, fibroids are a common finding and it is unnecessary to remove them simply to avoid malignant change in the future. There is also no evidence that a larger fibroid is more likely to become malignant, which means that size is not an indication for removal. An algorithm for the clinical management of fibroids is depicted in Figure 7.3. As long as the ultrasound scan reveals a normal fibroid with no changes suggestive of malignancy or degeneration, then the only reason to treat is on the basis of symptoms.

Clearly this presents a problem for the practitioner, as it is important to be certain that the patient's symptoms can be attributed to the fibroid and are not an incidental finding. It is not uncommon for symptoms that have been attributed to fibroids, such as backache, to continue after successful treatment of the tumor.

Although the subject of much discussion, there is no confirmatory evidence that fibroids cause infertility apart from when they obstruct the fallopian tubes at the cornu or distort adnexal anatomic relationships. Consequently, there are few indications for surgical removal of a fibroid to improve future fertility. In view of the possible complications of surgery, particularly tubal damage and loss of integrity of the endometrial cavity, such treatment should be considered only in rare circumstances.

Treatment of fibroids

A number of treatment options may be considered (Table 7.1).

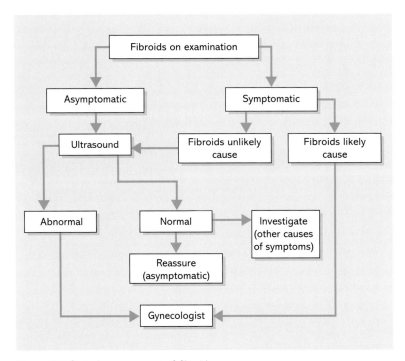

Figure 7.3 Clinical management of fibroids.

TABLE 7.1

Treatment of fibroids

Medical	Surgical
• Oral contraceptives	• Myomectomy
• NSAIDs	• Hysteroscopic resection
• GnRH agonists	• Hysterectomy

Interventional radiology
• Uterine artery embolization

Medical treatment is indicated for those women who wish to have further pregnancies. It is unlikely to be as effective as surgical treatment but can be used temporarily.

Oral contraceptives will decrease the menstrual loss in some women with fibroids, whether or not fibroids are the cause of the problem. Oral contraceptives have also been shown to have a protective effect on the growth of fibroids; they are, therefore, particularly useful in young women wishing future fertility, especially if they also require contraception.

NSAIDs will decrease menstrual loss in some women although this effect is likely to be small if the fibroids are the cause of the problem.

GnRH agonists are an effective treatment of fibroids because they induce a hypo-estrogenic state (discussed previously). The removal of the estrogen stimulation leads to shrinkage of the fibroid by as much as 50% after 2 months' therapy. GnRH agonists also induce amenorrhea, which is very helpful for women with DUB. There is no doubt that this form of therapy is effective in shrinking the fibroid and reducing symptoms; however, it is expensive and the attendant bone demineralization limits its use to 6 months.

GnRH agonists are likely to have three main indications:
• the perimenopausal woman
• prior to myomectomy
• prior to hysterectomy.

The perimenopausal woman may benefit from treatment with GnRH agonists because the fibroids will be treated effectively, and by the end of therapy she may have undergone the menopause. This avoids the need for major surgery. The shrinkage that GnRH agonists effect may make both myomectomy and hysterectomy easier to perform. This is especially true if the fibroid is in a difficult position, say within the cervix. The preoperative treatment also has the benefit of relieving the symptoms, and will treat anemia by inducing amenorrhea. Currently there is considerable debate on whether the benefit to both the surgeon and the patient justifies the cost of the treatment.

Interventional radiology

Uterine artery embolization has been used worldwide to treat patients with pain and menorrhagia secondary to leiomyoma. Although approximately 3–5% of women require additional treatment, overall the method is safe and effective for those who desire a less invasive management.

Surgical treatment

Myomectomy is surgical removal of the fibroid. The main indication is when there is a symptomatic fibroid and the woman wishes further pregnancies. Considerable technical difficulties may be associated with the operation and occasionally a hysterectomy has to be performed because of uncontrolled bleeding. This complication has been limited by the preoperative use of GnRH agonists. The difficulty and length of the operation, however, may mean that the tubes and ovaries are damaged either directly or through the desiccation of tissue that occurs during an open abdominal procedure. With these attendant problems, it is mandatory that the clinician is sure that the fibroid is the cause of the problem and that its removal will benefit the patient.

Hysteroscopic resection. If the fibroid is submucosal it can be resected through a hysteroscope. This can be performed as a day-case procedure and causes less discomfort to the patient. Evaluation of this technique is currently taking place. Exactly the same restrictions as discussed above are relevant for hysteroscopic resection. There is no evidence yet that such a resection improves fertility. Some authorities have discussed the possibility that removal of a submucosal fibroid will treat recurrent miscarriage, although confirmatory evidence is lacking. In addition, an abnormal endometrial cavity will be left at the end of the procedure. Studies on whether it is the removal of the fibroid or the endometrial resection that treats DUB are currently under way. It is important to stress that this is a skilled technique and there is considerable potential for damage if performed incorrectly. At present, family physicians should wait for more objective data before recommending it to their patients.

Hysterectomy. There is no doubt that hysterectomy will solve the problems of fibroids. Again, the clinician should be certain that the fibroid is the cause of the problem. The effectiveness of the procedure means that it is the yardstick against which all other techniques should be judged.

Key references

Braude P, Reidy J, Nott V et al. Embolization of uterine leiomyomata: current concepts in management. *Hum Reprod Update* 2000;6:603–8.

Brunereau L, Herbreteau D, Gallas S et al. Uterine artery embolization in the primary treatment of uterine leiomyomas: technical features and prospective follow-up with clinical and sonographic examinations in 58 patients. *Am J Roentgenol* 2000;175: 1267–72.

Stones RW. Uterine fibroids. In: Stones RW, ed. *Gynaecology Highlights 2000–01*. Oxford: Health Press Limited, 2001:42–50.

Vercellini P, Maddalena S, De Giorgi O et al. Determinants of reproductive outcome after abdominal myomectomy for infertility. *Fertil Steril* 1999;72:109–14.

Vercellini P, Zaina B, Yaylayan L et al. Hysteroscopic myomectomy: long-term effects on menstrual pattern and fertility. *Obstet Gynecol* 1999;94:341–7.

Young AE, Malinak LR, Harper A et al. Uterine artery embolization for the treatment of symptomatic leiomyomata. *Obstet Gynecol* 2000;95:S26.

Vaginitis is a common gynecological problem encountered by family physicians and is a source of physical and emotional distress for patients. In some instances it is a frustration for physicians, particularly if there is recurrent or chronic disease. Unfortunately, management is sometimes difficult because of the use of a wide variety of self-administered vaginal preparations.

The vaginal ecosystem depends on the balance of endogenous microflora and their metabolic products, the patient's level of estrogen and the vaginal pH level. This equilibrium may be challenged by endogenous or exogenous factors. Vaginitis usually occurs when the balance has been altered by factors such as medication, douching or other self-treatment. For example, antibiotics may allow the overgrowth of yeast and may suppress the growth of commensal organisms. Douching may alter the pH level or suppress the growth of endogenous bacteria.

Maintaining a normal pH level (3.8–4.2) stabilizes the vagina. pH levels are maintained in the normal range by *Lactobacillus acidophilus*, which is the dominant bacterium in a healthy vaginal environment. *Lactobacillus* spp. suppress the growth of pathogens and obligate anaerobes, thus maintaining a normal pH through the production of lactic acid.

Careful examination of the vagina with close inspection of the external genitalia is of paramount importance. It is necessary to establish whether symptoms arise from the vulva or vagina or both. Having established that the vagina is involved, alterations in the environment can be determined by identifying the gross and microscopic characteristics of the vaginal discharge. Vaginitis may exist in a number of different forms.

Bacterial vaginosis

Pathogenesis. Bacterial vaginosis (BV) which was previously known as non-specific vaginitis, results from the replacement of aerobic, hydrogen peroxide-producing lactobacilli normally found in the vagina with high concentrations of anaerobic and other bacteria, such as:

- *Gardnerella vaginalis*
- *Mobiluncus* spp.
- *Mycoplasma hominis*
- *Ureaplasma urealyticum*
- *Prevotella bivius*
- various *Bacteroides* spp.
- *Peptostreptococcus* spp.

Many of these microflora, such as *G. vaginalis* and *M. hominis*, may be found in healthy women but in lower concentrations; whereas others, such as *Mobiluncus mulieris*, are associated exclusively with BV. It has been reported that the intestine acts as a reservoir for BV microorganisms and also that male partners with such organisms in the proximal urethra may play a role in inoculating and reinfecting susceptible women.

The prevalence of BV in sexually active women is approximately 10–40%; approximately 50% of women with BV are asymptomatic. Several mechanisms have been suggested as possible contributory factors for the development of the disease including:

- retention of a diaphragm or tampon
- recent IUD placement
- administration of *Lactobacillus*-depleting antibiotics
- multiple sexual partners.

Investigations. Patients with BV have a homogeneous, white, non-inflammatory, milky, malodorous fishy discharge that adheres to the vaginal walls. The odor results from the metabolic by-products of anaerobic bacteria. Interestingly, vulval pruritus is not a common symptom. A 'whiff test' should be conducted, in which a drop of vaginal discharge is placed on a glass slide and a drop of 10% potassium hydroxide (KOH) added. If anaerobic bacteria are present, a fishy odor of amines will be noted. A wet-mount microscopic examination will reveal clue cells. Gram stain will reveal an abundance of bacteria of various morphologies. The pH level should be measured by placing pH paper on the lateral vaginal wall or immersing the strip in vaginal discharge. A pH greater than 4.5 will be indicated in BV. Diagnosis is established by finding three of the four signs indicated in Table 8.1.

Management. There are two topical vaginal regimens available for the treatment of BV: metronidazole and clindamycin (Table 8.2). Oral regimens of these two antimicrobial agents are equally effective.

TABLE 8.1

Clinical manifestations of bacterial vaginosis

- Homogeneous, white, non-inflammatory milky, malodorous fishy discharge that adheres to vaginal walls
- Vaginal pH > 4.5
- Positive whiff test
- Presence of clue cells on wet-mount microscopic examination

---

TABLE 8.2

Treatment of bacterial vaginosis

First-line
- Metronidazole, 400 mg orally twice daily for 7 days

Alternative regimens
- Clindamycin cream, 2%, one full applicator, intravaginally at bedtime for 7 days
- Clindamycin 300 mg orally twice daily for 7 days
- Metronidazole, 2 g orally in a single dose

Pregnant patients
- Clindamycin cream, 2%, one full applicator intravaginally at bedtime for 7 days during 1st trimester
- Metronidazole is contraindicated for use in 1st trimester
- During the 2nd and 3rd trimesters oral metronidazole can be used, but clindamycin cream or metronidazole gel is preferred

Treatment of the male partner is controversial. Most studies have not demonstrated an improved cure rate with the treatment of the partner at the first episode. Patients with recurrent BV should be screened for other venereal diseases.

Vulvovaginal candidiasis

Pathogenesis. *Candida* spp. can be identified on routine microscopic examination of vaginal discharge in approximately 30% of women with a healthy vaginal environment. These patients may be asymptomatic and require no treatment. However, certain factors may change this, such that proliferation and invasion of *Candida* spp. may result in the patient developing vaginal itching and burning. Approximately 15–30% of all vulvovaginal infections are caused by *Candida* spp. Most are caused by *C. albicans*, but other species such as *C. tropicalis* and *C. glabrata* play an increasingly prominent role in the etiology of this disease.

Numerous factors can predispose a woman to develop vulvovaginal candidiasis (VVC), including certain diseases or other physiologic changes such as:

- Cushing's or Addison's disease
- poorly controlled diabetes mellitus
- pregnancy
- vaginal trauma.

Certain drugs, contraceptive methods and lifestyle practices may also be implicated, such as:

- broad-spectrum antibiotics
- hormone therapy
- radiotherapy/chemotherapy
- tight-fitting synthetic underwear.

Investigations. Patients with VVC may develop both vaginal itching and vulval burning. Typically the vaginal discharge does not smell and is white with a 'cottage cheese-like' consistency that adheres to the vaginal walls. The vagina is usually hyperemic and excoriations may be noted on the vulva due to scratching or contact irritation. pH is not usually altered in VVC. Microscopic examination of vaginal discharge diluted with saline (wet-mount) and 10% KOH preparations will reveal hyphal forms or budding yeast cells in over half of patients. Over-the-counter non-specific and antifungal agents may mask other causes of vaginitis or select for resistant strains of yeast. It is important to ask the patient to discontinue use of such medications at least 72 hours before examination.

Management. VVC may be treated with broad-spectrum topical azoles (Table 8.3). Their effectiveness is believed to be due to the elimination of the rectal reservoir of yeast. Treatment of male partners is usually not necessary, though if he has symptoms of yeast balanitis or is uncircumcised, he may be a source of reinfection and should be treated.

Trichomoniasis

Pathogenesis. Trichomoniasis, caused by the organism *Trichomonas vaginalis*, is one of the most common sexually transmitted diseases and the third leading cause of vaginitis. The incidence of the disease, however, has steadily declined over the past two decades and several factors account for this trend:

- an increased understanding of the disease
- improved diagnostic techniques
- more effective therapy
- treatment of sexual partners.

Some reports indicate that trichomoniasis is more common in older women than in those in their teens, with the predominant occurrence being in women aged 20–29 years. It is particularly prevalent in women with multiple sexual partners.

Investigations. The clinical symptoms of trichomoniasis vary widely from patient to patient and range from an absence of symptoms in about 15% of women to severe, acute inflammatory disease in others. However, about one third of asymptomatic female carriers become symptomatic within 6 months. The common symptoms include a copious yellow-grey or green homogeneous, malodorous discharge. Vulvovaginal irritation and, on occasion, dysuria may also be present.

TABLE 8.3

Treatment of vulvovaginal candidiasis

Broad-spectrum topical azoles
- Terconazole*
  - 80 mg suppository for 3 days
  - 0.8% cream 5 g intravaginally for 3 days
  - 0.4% cream 5 g intravaginally for 7 days
- Butoconazole nitrate*
  - 2% cream 5 g intravaginally for 3 days
- Clotrimazole
  - 1% cream 5 g intravaginally for 7–14 days
  - 100 mg vaginal tablet for 7 days
  - 500 mg vaginal tablet in a single application
- Fluconazole
  - 150 mg orally in a single dose
- Miconazole nitrate
  - 2% cream, 1 full applicator, twice daily intravaginally for 7 days
  - 100 mg vaginal suppository, 1 suppository for 7 days
  - 200 mg vaginal suppository, 1 suppository for 3 days
- Tioconazole*
  - 6.5% ointment 5 g intravaginally in a single application

Pregnant patients

Topical therapies only, 7-day regimen
(clotrimazole, miconazole, butoconazole, and terconazole)

Chronic/recurrent infection of mild-to-moderate VVC

Fluconazole 150 mg capsule in a single dose

*Not available in the UK at time of press

The pH level of the discharge is usually greater than 4.5. Patients may also have a frothy discharge and/or a 'strawberry' or ecchymotic cervix. The diagnosis of a trichomonal infection is confirmed by examining a fresh wet-mount for mobile flagellated organisms. Occasionally, the diagnosis may be established on the results of a cervical smear test without the use of wet-mount.

Management. Standard treatment for trichomoniasis is metronidazole; sexual partners must be treated simultaneously for treatment to be effective (Table 8.4). Patients should be advised to avoid sex or use a condom until both they and their partner(s) are cured. Resistant trichomonal infections are rare but should be treated with higher doses of metronidazole (2.5 g per day) combined with intravaginal metronidazole suppositories (500 mg once or twice daily) for 10 days.

TABLE 8.4

Treatment of trichomoniasis

First-line
Metronidazole, 2 g orally in a single dose

Alternative regimens
Metronidazole, 500 mg orally twice daily for 7 days
Metronidazole, 250 mg orally three times daily for 7 days

Pregnant patients
Metronidazole is contraindicated in the 1st trimester
After the 1st trimester patients may be treated with 2 g metronidazole in a single oral dose

Key references

Vaginitis. *Technical Bulletin of the American College of Obstetricians and Gynecologists*, No. 221. March 1996.

Vulvovaginitis: A practice protocol for the managed care clinician. *National Association of Managed Care Physicians Round Table Highlights*. Gardiner Caldwell SynerMed 1996;1:1.

Warner P, Bancroft J. Factors related to self-reporting of the premenstrual syndrome. *Br J Psychiatry* 1990;157: 249–60.

Benign gynecological disease, particularly menstrual disorder, is the most common reason for a woman to consult her family physician or her gynecologist. The impact these conditions have on women's health and subsequent economic and social functioning will be increasingly recognized in the future. Inevitably their importance in future health policy will become greater. The size of the problem alone should justify increased research funding – a change that has occurred in the USA but not to such an extent in the UK as yet. Such research, especially into the biology of diseases such as endometriosis and fibroids, should provide a more rational basis for diagnosis and treatment.

There is an increasing realization that benign gynecological diseases are not necessarily abnormal conditions. Indeed, many are simply a manifestation of the extremes of normality. For example, nearly half of women complaining of heavy periods have a normal loss when measured objectively. Mild endometriosis may be a very common finding in many women and of no significance in the majority. Social changes mean that women experience many more menses in a reproductive life compared with the hunter–gatherer state in which both pregnancy and lactational amenorrhea limited menses. Complaints about menstrual disorders may reflect the order of magnitude of change in exposure. A clearer recognition of this by both women and practitioners will lead to different and possibly less interventionist strategies in the future.

Perhaps the biggest area for change over the next 10 years will be the relative roles of surgical versus medical treatment of these problems. There can be no doubt that surgery is an effective modality but it is invasive, with some risks, and many patients are wary of it. There are social changes that mean women are less likely to accept that the correct approach is to deprive them of their reproductive inheritance. However, while many medical therapies are effective, there are unacceptable side-effects for many women and that, combined with their expense, makes long-term use untenable. A number of compounds, particularly anti-estrogens that may be tissue selective or able to suppress plasma estradiol concentrations to just above menopausal levels, are currently being evaluated in Phase I and II studies. Nevertheless, they are still a long way from being considered successful and cheap therapeutic options. Therapies resulting from molecular and cellular studies of the endometrium and the ovary are still only in the earliest stages of development. There are exciting possibilities, such as gene transfer to the endometrium in order to control its proliferation. We await these developments with interest.

There is a general movement in all specialties towards evidence-based medicine and this is particularly true in primary care, where treatment protocols are evolving. Initial treatment may be by nurse–telephone triage and by mid-level providers such as nurse practitioners and physicians' assistants. Eventually 'internet consultations' with a 'real-time' televideo examination will avoid a trip to the doctor. Whatever happens, these changes in the understanding of menstrual disorders will mean that therapeutic choice will be a collaborative decision between women and their medical attendants. Surgery to alleviate normal menses which adversely affect a woman's life is not illogical. However, it is only right and proper that the patient understands that this option is not curative, and is aware of the risks involved. While the tools at our disposal may not change radically, the timing and the way in which we use them may be unrecognizable in 10 years' time.

Index

67